THIS JOURNAL BELONGS TO:

_____

_____

_____

- INTRODUCTION -

Are you ready to let plants rock your world? Take the next 90 days and increase the amount of fruits & vegetables in your diet - you'll be amazed with the results!

Use this food log and journal to track your daily servings of whole grains, beans & legumes, berries and other fruits, cruciferous vegetables, greens, nuts and seeds. Power Up your health with additional servings, track your hydration, and keep track of how you feel.

Look for ways to knock out a number of servings in one meal - like a large salad with greens, beans, fruit and nuts - BAM! Add hummus instead of mayo to a veggie sandwich and there's another serving of beans.

So what exactly is a serving? Great Question! Use the following guidelines to figure out servings for each category.

Whole Grains:
1/2 cup hot cereal or cooked grains, pasta, or corn kernels; 1 tortilla or slice of bread; 1 cup cold cereal; 3 cups popped popcorn; 1/2 a bagel or 1 English muffin

Beans:
1/4 cup hummus or bean dip; 1 cup of fresh peas or sprouted lentils; 1/2 cup cooked beans, split peas, lentils, tofu, or tempeh.

Berries:
1/2 cup fresh or frozen; 1/4 cup dried

Other Fruits:
1 medium-sized fruit; 1 cup cut up fruit; 1/4 cup dried fruit

Greens:
1 cup raw; 1/2 cup cooked

Cruciferous Vegetables:
1/2 cup chopped; 1/4 cup brussels or broccoli sprouts; 1 tablespoon horseradish

Other Vegetables:
1 cup raw leafy vegetables; 1/2 cup raw or cooked non-leafy vegetables; 1/2 cup vegetable juice; 1/4 cup dried mushrooms

Flaxseed & Walnuts:
1 tablespoon flaxseed; 1/4 cup walnuts;

Other Nuts & Seeds:
1/4 cup nuts or seeds; 2 tablespoons nut or seed butter

"Let food be
thy medicine
and medicine
be thy food."
— Hippocrates

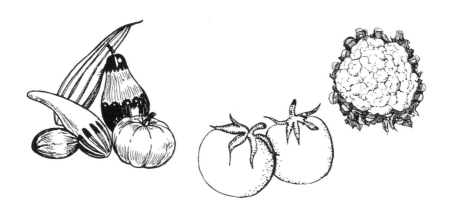

My Health Goals

	Starting #	Goal
Weight		
BMI		
Total Cholesterol		
Triglycerides		
LDL		
HDL		
Blood Pressure		
Blood Sugar H1AC		

Fitness Progress Tracker

What to Track	Week 1	Week 2
Weight		
Chest		
Hips		
Arms		
Thighs		

What to Track	Week 3	Week 4	Week 5	Week 6
Weight				
Chest				
Hips				
Arms				
Thighs				

What to Track	Week 7	Week 8	Week 8	Week 10
Weight				
Chest				
Hips				
Arms				
Thighs				

What to Track	Week 11	Week 12	Week 13	Week 14
Weight				
Chest				
Hips				
Arms				
Thighs				

Date: _____

	Daily Servings	Hunger / Cravings

Whole Grains ☐ ☐ ☐ ☐

Beans & Legumes ☐ ☐ ☐

Berries ☐ ☐

Other Fruits ☐ ☐

Greens ☐ ☐

Cruciferous Vegetables ☐

Other Vegetables ☐

Flaxseed & Walnuts ☐

Other Nuts & Seeds ☐

Hunger / Cravings

Some
None   Intense

Hydration

My Favorite Meal / Recipe Today Was:

_____

_____

_____

_____

_____

Today's Weight

Notes / My Important Numbers:

_____

_____

_____

_____

_____

_____

_____

Today I Feel...

Sleep Quality

Sleep Time

_____

Wake Time

_____

Date: _____

Daily Servings

🌾 Whole Grains ☐ ☐ ☐ ☐

🫘 Beans & Legumes ☐ ☐ ☐

🍓 Berries ☐ ☐

🍐 Other Fruits ☐ ☐

🥬 Greens ☐ ☐

🥦 Cruciferous Vegetables ☐

🥗 Other Vegetables ☐

🌰 Flaxseed & Walnuts ☐

🥜 Other Nuts & Seeds ☐

Hunger / Cravings

Hydration

My Favorite Meal / Recipe Today Was:

_____

_____

_____

_____

_____

Today's Weight

Notes / My Important Numbers:

_____

_____

_____

_____

_____

_____

_____

_____

Today I Feel...

Sleep Quality

Sleep Time

_____

Wake Time

_____

Date: _____

Daily Servings

🌾 Whole Grains ☐ ☐ ☐ ☐

🫘 Beans & Legumes ☐ ☐ ☐

🍓 Berries ☐ ☐

🍐 Other Fruits ☐ ☐

🥬 Greens ☐ ☐

🥦 Cruciferous Vegetables ☐

🍆 Other Vegetables ☐

🌰 Flaxseed & Walnuts ☐

🥜 Other Nuts & Seeds ☐

Hunger / Cravings

None · Some · Intense

Hydration

My Favorite Meal / Recipe Today Was:

_____

_____

_____

_____

_____

Today's Weight

Notes / My Important Numbers:

_____

_____

_____

_____

_____

_____

_____

Today I Feel...

Sleep Quality

Sleep Time

_____

Wake Time

_____

Date: _____

Daily Servings

🌾 Whole Grains ☐ ☐ ☐ ☐

🫘 Beans & Legumes ☐ ☐ ☐

🍓 Berries ☐ ☐

🍏 Other Fruits ☐ ☐

🥬 Greens ☐ ☐

🥦 Cruciferous Vegetables ☐

🥕 Other Vegetables ☐

🌰 Flaxseed & Walnuts ☐

🥜 Other Nuts & Seeds ☐

Hunger / Cravings

Some

None   Intense

Hydration

My Favorite Meal / Recipe Today Was:

_____

_____

_____

_____

Today's Weight

Notes / My Important Numbers:

_____

_____

_____

_____

_____

_____

_____

Today I Feel...

Sleep Quality

Sleep Time

_____

Wake Time

_____

Date: _____

Daily Servings

🌾 Whole Grains ☐ ☐ ☐ ☐

🫘 Beans & Legumes ☐ ☐ ☐

🍓 Berries ☐ ☐

🍑 Other Fruits ☐ ☐

🥬 Greens ☐ ☐

🥦 Cruciferous Vegetables ☐

🥕 Other Vegetables ☐

🌰 Flaxseed & Walnuts ☐

🥜 Other Nuts & Seeds ☐

Hunger / Cravings

Some

None · Intense

Hydration

My Favorite Meal / Recipe Today Was:

_____
_____
_____
_____
_____

Today's Weight

Notes / My Important Numbers:

_____
_____
_____
_____
_____
_____
_____
_____

Today I Feel...

Sleep Quality

Sleep Time

_____

Wake Time

_____

Date: _____

		Daily Servings	Hunger / Cravings

Whole Grains ☐ ☐ ☐ ☐

Beans & Legumes ☐ ☐ ☐

Berries ☐ ☐

Other Fruits ☐ ☐

Greens ☐ ☐

Cruciferous Vegetables ☐

Other Vegetables ☐

Flaxseed & Walnuts ☐

Other Nuts & Seeds ☐

Hunger / Cravings

Some

None — Intense

Hydration

My Favorite Meal / Recipe Today Was:

_____

_____

_____

_____

_____

Today's Weight

Notes / My Important Numbers:

_____

_____

_____

_____

_____

_____

_____

Today I Feel...

Sleep Quality

Sleep Time

_____

Wake Time

_____

Date: _____

	Daily Servings	

🌾 Whole Grains ☐ ☐ ☐ ☐

🫘 Beans & Legumes ☐ ☐ ☐

🍓 Berries ☐ ☐

🍐 Other Fruits ☐ ☐

🥦 Greens ☐ ☐

🥦 Cruciferous Vegetables ☐

🥕 Other Vegetables ☐

🌰 Flaxseed & Walnuts ☐

🥜 Other Nuts & Seeds ☐

Hunger / Cravings

Some

None — Intense

Hydration

My Favorite Meal / Recipe Today Was:

_____
_____
_____
_____
_____

Today's Weight

Notes / My Important Numbers:

_____
_____
_____
_____
_____
_____
_____
_____

Today I Feel...

Sleep Quality

Sleep Time

_____

Wake Time

_____

Date: _____

Daily Servings

- 🌾 Whole Grains ☐ ☐ ☐ ☐
- 🫘 Beans & Legumes ☐ ☐ ☐
- 🍓 Berries ☐ ☐
- 🍐 Other Fruits ☐ ☐
- 🥬 Greens ☐ ☐
- 🥦 Cruciferous Vegetables ☐
- 🥕 Other Vegetables ☐
- 🌿 Flaxseed & Walnuts ☐
- 🥜 Other Nuts & Seeds ☐

Hunger / Cravings

Hydration

My Favorite Meal / Recipe Today Was:

_____
_____
_____
_____
_____

Today's Weight

Notes / My Important Numbers:

_____
_____
_____
_____
_____
_____
_____
_____

Today I Feel...

Sleep Quality

Sleep Time
_____

Wake Time
_____

Date: _____

Daily Servings

- 🌾 Whole Grains ☐ ☐ ☐ ☐
- 🫘 Beans & Legumes ☐ ☐ ☐
- 🍓 Berries ☐ ☐
- 🍐 Other Fruits ☐ ☐
- 🥬 Greens ☐ ☐
- 🥦 Cruciferous Vegetables ☐
- 🥕 Other Vegetables ☐
- 🌰 Flaxseed & Walnuts ☐
- 🥜 Other Nuts & Seeds ☐

Hunger / Cravings

Some

None   Intense

Hydration

My Favorite Meal / Recipe Today Was:

_____
_____
_____
_____

Today's Weight

Notes / My Important Numbers:

_____
_____
_____
_____
_____
_____
_____

Today I Feel...

Sleep Quality

Sleep Time
_____

Wake Time
_____

Date: _____

	Daily Servings	Hunger / Cravings

Whole Grains ☐ ☐ ☐ ☐

Beans & Legumes ☐ ☐ ☐

Berries ☐ ☐

Other Fruits ☐ ☐

Greens ☐ ☐

Cruciferous Vegetables ☐

Other Vegetables ☐

Flaxseed & Walnuts ☐

Other Nuts & Seeds ☐

Hunger / Cravings

Some

None — Intense

Hydration

My Favorite Meal / Recipe Today Was:

_____

_____

_____

_____

_____

Today's Weight

Notes / My Important Numbers:

_____

_____

_____

_____

_____

_____

_____

Today I Feel...

Sleep Quality

Sleep Time

_____

Wake Time

_____

Date: _____

Daily Servings

🌾 Whole Grains	☐ ☐ ☐ ☐
🫘 Beans & Legumes	☐ ☐ ☐
🍓 Berries	☐ ☐
🍑 Other Fruits	☐ ☐
🥦 Greens	☐ ☐
🥦 Cruciferous Vegetables	☐
🥕 Other Vegetables	☐
🌰 Flaxseed & Walnuts	☐
🥜 Other Nuts & Seeds	☐

Hunger / Cravings

Some
None
Intense

Hydration

My Favorite Meal / Recipe Today Was:

_____
_____
_____
_____
_____

Today's Weight

Notes / My Important Numbers:

_____
_____
_____
_____
_____
_____
_____

Today I Feel...

Sleep Quality

Sleep Time

_____

Wake Time

_____

Date: _____

		Daily Servings

Whole Grains ☐ ☐ ☐ ☐

Beans & Legumes ☐ ☐ ☐

Berries ☐ ☐

Other Fruits ☐ ☐

Greens ☐ ☐

Cruciferous Vegetables ☐

Other Vegetables ☐

Flaxseed & Walnuts ☐

Other Nuts & Seeds ☐

Hunger / Cravings

Some

None   Intense

Hydration

My Favorite Meal / Recipe Today Was:

_____

_____

_____

_____

_____

Today's Weight

Notes / My Important Numbers:

_____

_____

_____

_____

_____

_____

_____

_____

Today I Feel...

Sleep Quality

Sleep Time

_____

Wake Time

_____

Date: _____

	Daily Servings	Hunger / Cravings

Daily Servings

🌾 Whole Grains   ☐ ☐ ☐ ☐

🫘 Beans & Legumes   ☐ ☐ ☐

🍓 Berries   ☐ ☐

🍐 Other Fruits   ☐ ☐

🥦 Greens   ☐ ☐

🥦 Cruciferous Vegetables   ☐

🥕 Other Vegetables   ☐

🌰 Flaxseed & Walnuts   ☐

🫘 Other Nuts & Seeds   ☐

Hunger / Cravings

Some

None   Intense

Hydration

My Favorite Meal / Recipe Today Was:

_____

_____

_____

_____

_____

Today's Weight

Notes / My Important Numbers:

_____

_____

_____

_____

_____

_____

_____

Today I Feel...

Sleep Quality

Sleep Time

_____

Wake Time

_____

Date: _____

		Daily Servings			

Whole Grains ☐ ☐ ☐ ☐

Beans & Legumes ☐ ☐ ☐

Berries ☐ ☐

Other Fruits ☐ ☐

Greens ☐ ☐

Cruciferous Vegetables ☐

Other Vegetables ☐

Flaxseed & Walnuts ☐

Other Nuts & Seeds ☐

Hunger / Cravings

Some
None   Intense

Hydration

My Favorite Meal / Recipe Today Was:

_____
_____
_____
_____
_____

Today's Weight

Notes / My Important Numbers:

_____
_____
_____
_____
_____
_____
_____

Today I Feel...

Sleep Quality

Sleep Time

_____

Wake Time

_____

Date: _____

Whole Grains ☐ ☐ ☐ ☐

Beans & Legumes ☐ ☐ ☐

Berries ☐ ☐

Other Fruits ☐ ☐

Greens ☐ ☐

Cruciferous Vegetables ☐

Other Vegetables ☐

Flaxseed & Walnuts ☐

Other Nuts & Seeds ☐

Hunger / Cravings

Some

None   Intense

Hydration

My Favorite Meal / Recipe Today Was:

_____
_____
_____
_____

Today's Weight

Notes / My Important Numbers:

_____
_____
_____
_____
_____
_____
_____

Today I Feel...

Sleep Quality

Sleep Time
_____

Wake Time
_____

Date: _____

		Daily Servings	Hunger / Cravings

Whole Grains ☐ ☐ ☐ ☐

Beans & Legumes ☐ ☐ ☐

Berries ☐ ☐

Other Fruits ☐ ☐

Greens ☐ ☐

Cruciferous Vegetables ☐

Other Vegetables ☐

Flaxseed & Walnuts ☐

Other Nuts & Seeds ☐

Daily Servings

Hunger / Cravings

Some
None   Intense

Hydration

My Favorite Meal / Recipe Today Was:

_____

_____

_____

_____

_____

Today's Weight

Notes / My Important Numbers:

_____

_____

_____

_____

_____

_____

_____

Today I Feel...

Sleep Quality

Sleep Time
_____

Wake Time
_____

Date: _____

| | Daily Servings | Hunger / Cravings |

Daily Servings

🌾 Whole Grains ☐ ☐ ☐ ☐

🫘 Beans & Legumes ☐ ☐ ☐

🍓 Berries ☐ ☐

🍐 Other Fruits ☐ ☐

🥦 Greens ☐ ☐

🥬 Cruciferous Vegetables ☐

🥕 Other Vegetables ☐

🌰 Flaxseed & Walnuts ☐

🥜 Other Nuts & Seeds ☐

Hunger / Cravings

Some

None · Intense

Hydration

My Favorite Meal / Recipe Today Was:

_____

_____

_____

Today's Weight

Notes / My Important Numbers:

_____

_____

_____

_____

_____

_____

_____

Today I Feel...

Sleep Quality

Sleep Time

_____

Wake Time

_____

Date: _____

Daily Servings

🌾 Whole Grains   ☐ ☐ ☐ ☐

🫘 Beans & Legumes   ☐ ☐ ☐

🍓 Berries   ☐ ☐

🍐 Other Fruits   ☐ ☐

🥬 Greens   ☐ ☐

🥦 Cruciferous Vegetables   ☐

🥗 Other Vegetables   ☐

🌰 Flaxseed & Walnuts   ☐

🥜 Other Nuts & Seeds   ☐

Hunger / Cravings

Some

None   Intense

Hydration

My Favorite Meal / Recipe Today Was:

_____
_____
_____
_____
_____

Today's Weight

Notes / My Important Numbers:

_____
_____
_____
_____
_____
_____
_____

Today I Feel...

Sleep Quality

Sleep Time

_____

Wake Time

_____

Date: _____

	Daily Servings			
🌾 Whole Grains	☐	☐	☐	☐
🫘 Beans & Legumes	☐	☐	☐	
🍓 Berries	☐	☐		
🍐 Other Fruits	☐	☐		
🥬 Greens	☐	☐		
🥦 Cruciferous Vegetables	☐			
🥕 Other Vegetables	☐			
🌰 Flaxseed & Walnuts	☐			
🥜 Other Nuts & Seeds	☐			

Hunger / Cravings

Some

None — Intense

Hydration

My Favorite Meal / Recipe Today Was:

_____

_____

_____

_____

_____

Today's Weight

Notes / My Important Numbers:

_____

_____

_____

_____

_____

_____

_____

_____

Today I Feel...

Sleep Quality

Sleep Time

_____

Wake Time

_____

Date: _____

Daily Servings

🌾 Whole Grains ☐ ☐ ☐ ☐

🫘 Beans & Legumes ☐ ☐ ☐

🍓 Berries ☐ ☐

🍐 Other Fruits ☐ ☐

🥬 Greens ☐ ☐

🥦 Cruciferous Vegetables ☐

🥗 Other Vegetables ☐

🌰 Flaxseed & Walnuts ☐

🥜 Other Nuts & Seeds ☐

Hunger / Cravings

Some
None   Intense

Hydration

My Favorite Meal / Recipe Today Was:

_____
_____
_____
_____

Today's Weight

Notes / My Important Numbers:

_____
_____
_____
_____
_____
_____
_____
_____

Today I Feel...

Sleep Quality

Sleep Time
_____

Wake Time
_____

Date: _____

Daily Servings

🌾 Whole Grains	☐ ☐ ☐ ☐	
🫘 Beans & Legumes	☐ ☐ ☐	
🍓 Berries	☐ ☐	
🍎 Other Fruits	☐ ☐	
🥬 Greens	☐ ☐	
🥦 Cruciferous Vegetables	☐	
🥕 Other Vegetables	☐	
🌰 Flaxseed & Walnuts	☐	
🥜 Other Nuts & Seeds	☐	

Hunger / Cravings

Some

None   Intense

Hydration

My Favorite Meal / Recipe Today Was:

_____
_____
_____
_____
_____

Today's Weight

Notes / My Important Numbers:

_____
_____
_____
_____
_____
_____
_____

Today I Feel...

Sleep Quality

Sleep Time

_____

Wake Time

_____

Date: _____

		Daily Servings
🌾	Whole Grains	☐ ☐ ☐ ☐
🫘	Beans & Legumes	☐ ☐ ☐
🍓	Berries	☐ ☐
🍐	Other Fruits	☐ ☐
🥦	Greens	☐ ☐
🥦	Cruciferous Vegetables	☐
🥕	Other Vegetables	☐
🌰	Flaxseed & Walnuts	☐
🥜	Other Nuts & Seeds	☐

Hunger / Cravings

None — Some — Intense

Hydration

My Favorite Meal / Recipe Today Was:

_____

_____

_____

_____

_____

Today's Weight

Notes / My Important Numbers:

_____

_____

_____

_____

_____

_____

_____

_____

Today I Feel...

Sleep Quality

Sleep Time

_____

Wake Time

_____

Date: _____

		Daily Servings			

Whole Grains ☐ ☐ ☐ ☐

Beans & Legumes ☐ ☐ ☐

Berries ☐ ☐

Other Fruits ☐ ☐

Greens ☐ ☐

Cruciferous Vegetables ☐

Other Vegetables ☐

Flaxseed & Walnuts ☐

Other Nuts & Seeds ☐

Hunger / Cravings

Some

None   Intense

Hydration

My Favorite Meal / Recipe Today Was:

_____

_____

_____

_____

Today's Weight

Notes / My Important Numbers:

_____

_____

_____

_____

_____

_____

_____

Today I Feel...

Sleep Quality

Sleep Time

_____

Wake Time

_____

Date: _____

		Daily Servings
🌾	Whole Grains	☐ ☐ ☐ ☐
🫘	Beans & Legumes	☐ ☐ ☐
🍓	Berries	☐ ☐
🍐	Other Fruits	☐ ☐
🥦	Greens	☐ ☐
🥦	Cruciferous Vegetables	☐
	Other Vegetables	☐
	Flaxseed & Walnuts	☐
	Other Nuts & Seeds	☐

Hunger / Cravings

Some

None   Intense

Hydration

My Favorite Meal / Recipe Today Was:

_____

_____

_____

_____

_____

Today's Weight

Notes / My Important Numbers:

_____

_____

_____

_____

_____

_____

_____

_____

Today I Feel...

Sleep Quality

Sleep Time

_____

Wake Time

_____

Date: _____

Daily Servings

Whole Grains ☐ ☐ ☐ ☐

Beans & Legumes ☐ ☐ ☐

Berries ☐ ☐

Other Fruits ☐ ☐

Greens ☐ ☐

Cruciferous Vegetables ☐

Other Vegetables ☐

Flaxseed & Walnuts ☐

Other Nuts & Seeds ☐

Hunger / Cravings

Hydration

My Favorite Meal / Recipe Today Was:

_____
_____
_____
_____

Today's Weight

Notes / My Important Numbers:

_____
_____
_____
_____
_____
_____
_____

Today I Feel...

Sleep Quality

Sleep Time
_____

Wake Time
_____

Date: _____

		Daily Servings	Hunger / Cravings

Whole Grains ☐ ☐ ☐ ☐

Beans & Legumes ☐ ☐ ☐

Berries ☐ ☐

Other Fruits ☐ ☐

Greens ☐ ☐

Cruciferous Vegetables ☐

Other Vegetables ☐

Flaxseed & Walnuts ☐

Other Nuts & Seeds ☐

Daily Servings

Hunger / Cravings

Some

None | Intense

Hydration

My Favorite Meal / Recipe Today Was:

_____

_____

_____

_____

_____

Today's Weight

Notes / My Important Numbers:

_____

_____

_____

_____

_____

_____

_____

_____

Today I Feel...

Sleep Quality

Sleep Time

_____

Wake Time

_____

Date: _____

	Daily Servings	Hunger / Cravings

Whole Grains ☐ ☐ ☐ ☐

Beans & Legumes ☐ ☐ ☐

Berries ☐ ☐

Other Fruits ☐ ☐

Greens ☐ ☐

Cruciferous Vegetables ☐

Other Vegetables ☐

Flaxseed & Walnuts ☐

Other Nuts & Seeds ☐

Hunger / Cravings

Some

None · Intense

Hydration

My Favorite Meal / Recipe Today Was:

_____

_____

_____

_____

Today's Weight

Notes / My Important Numbers:

_____

_____

_____

_____

_____

_____

_____

_____

Today I Feel...

Sleep Quality

Sleep Time

_____

Wake Time

_____

Date: _____

Whole Grains

Beans & Legumes

Berries

Other Fruits

Greens

Cruciferous Vegetables

Other Vegetables

Flaxseed & Walnuts

Other Nuts & Seeds

Daily Servings

Hunger / Cravings

Some

None

Intense

Hydration

My Favorite Meal / Recipe Today Was:

_____

_____

_____

_____

Today's Weight

Notes / My Important Numbers:

_____

_____

_____

_____

_____

_____

_____

_____

Today I Feel...

Sleep Quality

Sleep Time

_____

Wake Time

_____

Date: _____

Daily Servings

🌾 Whole Grains ☐ ☐ ☐ ☐

🫘 Beans & Legumes ☐ ☐ ☐

🍓 Berries ☐ ☐

🍐 Other Fruits ☐ ☐

🥦 Greens ☐ ☐

🥦 Cruciferous Vegetables ☐

🧅 Other Vegetables ☐

🌰 Flaxseed & Walnuts ☐

🥜 Other Nuts & Seeds ☐

Hunger / Cravings

Some

None   Intense

Hydration

My Favorite Meal / Recipe Today Was:

_____

_____

_____

_____

Today's Weight

Notes / My Important Numbers:

_____

_____

_____

_____

_____

_____

_____

Today I Feel...

Sleep Quality

Sleep Time

_____

Wake Time

_____

Date: _____

Daily Servings

Food	Servings
🌾 Whole Grains	☐ ☐ ☐ ☐
🫘 Beans & Legumes	☐ ☐ ☐
🍓 Berries	☐ ☐
🍎 Other Fruits	☐ ☐
🥬 Greens	☐ ☐
🥦 Cruciferous Vegetables	☐
🍆 Other Vegetables	☐
🌰 Flaxseed & Walnuts	☐
🥜 Other Nuts & Seeds	☐

Hunger / Cravings

Some

None — Intense

Hydration

My Favorite Meal / Recipe Today Was:

_____
_____
_____
_____
_____

Today's Weight

Notes / My Important Numbers:

_____
_____
_____
_____
_____
_____
_____
_____

Today I Feel...

Sleep Quality

Sleep Time

_____

Wake Time

_____

Date: _____

Hunger / Cravings

Whole Grains ☐ ☐ ☐ ☐

Beans & Legumes ☐ ☐ ☐

Berries ☐ ☐

Other Fruits ☐ ☐

Greens ☐ ☐

Cruciferous Vegetables ☐

Other Vegetables ☐

Flaxseed & Walnuts ☐

Other Nuts & Seeds ☐

Some

None

Intense

Hydration

My Favorite Meal / Recipe Today Was:

_____
_____
_____
_____

Today's Weight

Notes / My Important Numbers:

_____
_____
_____
_____
_____
_____
_____
_____

Today I Feel...

Sleep Quality

Sleep Time
_____

Wake Time
_____

Date: _____

Daily Servings

Food	Servings
🌾 Whole Grains	☐ ☐ ☐ ☐
🫘 Beans & Legumes	☐ ☐ ☐
🍓 Berries	☐ ☐
🍎 Other Fruits	☐ ☐
🥬 Greens	☐ ☐
🥦 Cruciferous Vegetables	☐
🥕 Other Vegetables	☐
🌰 Flaxseed & Walnuts	☐
🥜 Other Nuts & Seeds	☐

Hunger / Cravings

Some

None   Intense

Hydration

My Favorite Meal / Recipe Today Was:

_____

_____

_____

_____

_____

Today's Weight

Notes / My Important Numbers:

_____

_____

_____

_____

_____

_____

_____

_____

Today I Feel...

Sleep Quality

Sleep Time

_____

Wake Time

_____

Date: _____

Daily Servings

Whole Grains ☐ ☐ ☐ ☐

Beans & Legumes ☐ ☐ ☐

Berries ☐ ☐

Other Fruits ☐ ☐

Greens ☐ ☐

Cruciferous Vegetables ☐

Other Vegetables ☐

Flaxseed & Walnuts ☐

Other Nuts & Seeds ☐

Hunger / Cravings

Some
None   Intense

Hydration

My Favorite Meal / Recipe Today Was:

_____

_____

_____

_____

Today's Weight

Notes / My Important Numbers:

_____

_____

_____

_____

_____

_____

_____

Today I Feel...

Sleep Quality

Sleep Time

_____

Wake Time

_____

Date: _____

	Daily Servings	
Whole Grains	☐ ☐ ☐ ☐	
Beans & Legumes	☐ ☐ ☐	
Berries	☐ ☐	
Other Fruits	☐ ☐	
Greens	☐ ☐	
Cruciferous Vegetables	☐	
Other Vegetables	☐	
Flaxseed & Walnuts	☐	
Other Nuts & Seeds	☐	

Hunger / Cravings

Some

None   Intense

Hydration

My Favorite Meal / Recipe Today Was:

_____
_____
_____
_____
_____

Today's Weight

Notes / My Important Numbers:

_____
_____
_____
_____
_____
_____
_____
_____
_____

Today I Feel...

Sleep Quality

Sleep Time

_____

Wake Time

_____

Date: _____

	Daily Servings	
Whole Grains	☐ ☐ ☐ ☐	
Beans & Legumes	☐ ☐ ☐	
Berries	☐ ☐	
Other Fruits	☐ ☐	
Greens	☐ ☐	
Cruciferous Vegetables	☐	
Other Vegetables	☐	
Flaxseed & Walnuts	☐	
Other Nuts & Seeds	☐	

Hunger / Cravings

Some

None   Intense

Hydration

My Favorite Meal / Recipe Today Was:

_____

_____

_____

_____

Today's Weight

Notes / My Important Numbers:

_____

_____

_____

_____

_____

_____

_____

_____

Today I Feel...

Sleep Quality

Sleep Time

_____

Wake Time

_____

Date: _____

	Daily Servings	Hunger / Cravings

Whole Grains ☐ ☐ ☐ ☐

Beans & Legumes ☐ ☐ ☐

Berries ☐ ☐

Other Fruits ☐ ☐

Greens ☐ ☐

Cruciferous Vegetables ☐

Other Vegetables ☐

Flaxseed & Walnuts ☐

Other Nuts & Seeds ☐

Hunger / Cravings

None — Some — Intense

Hydration

My Favorite Meal / Recipe Today Was:

_____

_____

_____

_____

Today's Weight

Notes / My Important Numbers:

_____

_____

_____

_____

_____

_____

_____

_____

Today I Feel...

Sleep Quality

Sleep Time

_____

Wake Time

_____

Date: _____

Daily Servings

🌾 Whole Grains	☐ ☐ ☐ ☐	
🫘 Beans & Legumes	☐ ☐ ☐	
🍓 Berries	☐ ☐	
🍑 Other Fruits	☐ ☐	
🥬 Greens	☐ ☐	
🥦 Cruciferous Vegetables	☐	
🍅 Other Vegetables	☐	
🌰 Flaxseed & Walnuts	☐	
🥜 Other Nuts & Seeds	☐	

Hunger / Cravings

Some

None   Intense

Hydration

My Favorite Meal / Recipe Today Was:

_____

_____

_____

_____

_____

Today's Weight

Notes / My Important Numbers:

_____

_____

_____

_____

_____

_____

_____

_____

Today I Feel...

Sleep Quality

Sleep Time

_____

Wake Time

_____

Date: _____

Whole Grains
Beans & Legumes
Berries
Other Fruits
Greens
Cruciferous Vegetables
Other Vegetables
Flaxseed & Walnuts
Other Nuts & Seeds

Whole Grains
Beans & Legumes
Berries
Other Fruits
Greens
Cruciferous Vegetables
Other Vegetables
Flaxseed & Walnuts
Other Nuts & Seeds

Daily Servings

Hunger / Cravings

Some

None   Intense

Hydration

My Favorite Meal / Recipe Today Was:

_____
_____
_____
_____

Today's Weight

Notes / My Important Numbers:

_____
_____
_____
_____
_____
_____
_____

Today I Feel...

Sleep Quality

Sleep Time

_____

Wake Time

_____

Date: _____

Daily Servings

🌾	Whole Grains	☐ ☐ ☐ ☐
🫘	Beans & Legumes	☐ ☐ ☐
🍓	Berries	☐ ☐
🍑	Other Fruits	☐ ☐
🥦	Greens	☐ ☐
🥦	Cruciferous Vegetables	☐
🍅	Other Vegetables	☐
🌰	Flaxseed & Walnuts	☐
🥜	Other Nuts & Seeds	☐

Hunger / Cravings

Some

None   Intense

Hydration

My Favorite Meal / Recipe Today Was:

_____
_____
_____
_____

Today's Weight

Notes / My Important Numbers:

_____
_____
_____
_____
_____
_____
_____
_____

Today I Feel...

Sleep Quality

Sleep Time

_____

Wake Time

_____

Date: _____

	Daily Servings			
Whole Grains	☐	☐	☐	☐
Beans & Legumes	☐	☐	☐	
Berries	☐	☐		
Other Fruits	☐	☐		
Greens	☐	☐		
Cruciferous Vegetables	☐			
Other Vegetables	☐			
Flaxseed & Walnuts	☐			
Other Nuts & Seeds	☐			

Hunger / Cravings

Some

None

Intense

Hydration

My Favorite Meal / Recipe Today Was:

_____

_____

_____

_____

_____

Today's Weight

Notes / My Important Numbers:

_____

_____

_____

_____

_____

_____

_____

Today I Feel...

Sleep Quality

Sleep Time

_____

Wake Time

_____

Date: _____

Daily Servings

Food	Servings
🌾 Whole Grains	☐ ☐ ☐ ☐
🫘 Beans & Legumes	☐ ☐ ☐
🍓 Berries	☐ ☐
🍑 Other Fruits	☐ ☐
🥦 Greens	☐ ☐
🥦 Cruciferous Vegetables	☐
🥕 Other Vegetables	☐
🌰 Flaxseed & Walnuts	☐
🥜 Other Nuts & Seeds	☐

Hunger / Cravings

None — Some — Intense

Hydration

My Favorite Meal / Recipe Today Was:

_____
_____
_____
_____
_____

Today's Weight

Notes / My Important Numbers:

_____
_____
_____
_____
_____
_____
_____
_____

Today I Feel...

Sleep Quality

Sleep Time
_____

Wake Time
_____

Date: _____

		Daily Servings		Hunger / Cravings

Whole Grains ☐ ☐ ☐ ☐

Beans & Legumes ☐ ☐ ☐

Berries ☐ ☐

Other Fruits ☐ ☐

Greens ☐ ☐

Cruciferous Vegetables ☐

Other Vegetables ☐

Flaxseed & Walnuts ☐

Other Nuts & Seeds ☐

Daily Servings

Hunger / Cravings

Some

None — Intense

Hydration

My Favorite Meal / Recipe Today Was:

_____

_____

_____

_____

_____

Today's Weight

Notes / My Important Numbers:

_____

_____

_____

_____

_____

_____

_____

_____

Today I Feel...

Sleep Quality

Sleep Time

_____

Wake Time

_____

Date: _____

Daily Servings

Food	Servings
🌾 Whole Grains	☐ ☐ ☐ ☐
🫘 Beans & Legumes	☐ ☐ ☐
🍓 Berries	☐ ☐
🍐 Other Fruits	☐ ☐
🥬 Greens	☐ ☐
🥦 Cruciferous Vegetables	☐
🍅 Other Vegetables	☐
🌰 Flaxseed & Walnuts	☐
🥜 Other Nuts & Seeds	☐

Hunger / Cravings

Some
None — Intense

Hydration

My Favorite Meal / Recipe Today Was:

_____

_____

_____

_____

Today's Weight

Notes / My Important Numbers:

_____

_____

_____

_____

_____

_____

_____

Today I Feel...

Sleep Quality

Sleep Time

_____

Wake Time

_____

Date: _____

		Daily Servings	Hunger / Cravings

Whole Grains ☐ ☐ ☐ ☐

Beans & Legumes ☐ ☐ ☐

Berries ☐ ☐

Other Fruits ☐ ☐

Greens ☐ ☐

Cruciferous Vegetables ☐

Other Vegetables ☐

Flaxseed & Walnuts ☐

Other Nuts & Seeds ☐

Daily Servings

Hunger / Cravings

Some

None · Intense

Hydration

My Favorite Meal / Recipe Today Was:

_____

_____

_____

_____

_____

Today's Weight

Notes / My Important Numbers:

_____

_____

_____

_____

_____

_____

_____

_____

Today I Feel...

Sleep Quality

Sleep Time

_____

Wake Time

_____

Date: _____

Daily Servings

🌾 Whole Grains ☐ ☐ ☐ ☐

🫘 Beans & Legumes ☐ ☐ ☐

🍓 Berries ☐ ☐

🍐 Other Fruits ☐ ☐

🥬 Greens ☐ ☐

🥦 Cruciferous Vegetables ☐

🧅 Other Vegetables ☐

🥜 Flaxseed & Walnuts ☐

🌰 Other Nuts & Seeds ☐

Hunger / Cravings

Some

None

Intense

Hydration

My Favorite Meal / Recipe Today Was:

_____
_____
_____
_____
_____

Today's Weight

Notes / My Important Numbers:

_____
_____
_____
_____
_____
_____
_____
_____

Today I Feel...

Sleep Quality

Sleep Time
_____

Wake Time
_____

Date: _____

	Daily Servings	Hunger / Cravings

🌾 Whole Grains ☐ ☐ ☐ ☐

🫘 Beans & Legumes ☐ ☐ ☐

🍓 Berries ☐ ☐

🍐 Other Fruits ☐ ☐

🥬 Greens ☐ ☐

🥦 Cruciferous Vegetables ☐

🥗 Other Vegetables ☐

🌿 Flaxseed & Walnuts ☐

🥜 Other Nuts & Seeds ☐

Hunger / Cravings

Some · None · Intense

Hydration

My Favorite Meal / Recipe Today Was:

_____

_____

_____

_____

_____

Today's Weight

Notes / My Important Numbers:

_____

_____

_____

_____

_____

_____

_____

_____

Today I Feel...

Sleep Quality

Sleep Time

_____

Wake Time

_____

Date: _____

Hunger / Cravings

- Whole Grains ☐ ☐ ☐ ☐
- Beans & Legumes ☐ ☐ ☐
- Berries ☐ ☐
- Other Fruits ☐ ☐
- Greens ☐ ☐
- Cruciferous Vegetables ☐
- Other Vegetables ☐
- Flaxseed & Walnuts ☐
- Other Nuts & Seeds ☐

Some

None   Intense

Hydration

My Favorite Meal / Recipe Today Was:

_____
_____
_____
_____

Today's Weight

Notes / My Important Numbers:

_____
_____
_____
_____
_____
_____
_____

Today I Feel...

Sleep Quality

Sleep Time
_____

Wake Time
_____

Date: _____

		Daily Servings

Whole Grains ☐ ☐ ☐ ☐

Beans & Legumes ☐ ☐ ☐

Berries ☐ ☐

Other Fruits ☐ ☐

Greens ☐ ☐

Cruciferous Vegetables ☐

Other Vegetables ☐

Flaxseed & Walnuts ☐

Other Nuts & Seeds ☐

Hunger / Cravings

Some

None — Intense

Hydration

My Favorite Meal / Recipe Today Was:

_____

_____

_____

_____

Today's Weight

Notes / My Important Numbers:

_____

_____

_____

_____

_____

_____

_____

Today I Feel...

Sleep Quality

Sleep Time

_____

Wake Time

_____

Date: _____

Hunger / Cravings

Whole Grains ☐ ☐ ☐ ☐

Beans & Legumes ☐ ☐ ☐

Berries ☐ ☐

Other Fruits ☐ ☐

Greens ☐ ☐

Cruciferous Vegetables ☐

Other Vegetables ☐

Flaxseed & Walnuts ☐

Other Nuts & Seeds ☐

Some

None

Intense

Hydration

My Favorite Meal / Recipe Today Was:

_____

_____

_____

_____

_____

Today's Weight

Notes / My Important Numbers:

_____

_____

_____

_____

_____

_____

_____

Today I Feel...

Sleep Quality

Sleep Time

_____

Wake Time

_____

Date: _____

		Daily Servings	Hunger / Cravings

Whole Grains ☐ ☐ ☐ ☐

Beans & Legumes ☐ ☐ ☐

Berries ☐ ☐

Other Fruits ☐ ☐

Greens ☐ ☐

Cruciferous Vegetables ☐

Other Vegetables ☐

Flaxseed & Walnuts ☐

Other Nuts & Seeds ☐

Hunger / Cravings

Some / None / Intense

Hydration

My Favorite Meal / Recipe Today Was:

_____

_____

_____

_____

Today's Weight

Notes / My Important Numbers:

_____

_____

_____

_____

_____

_____

_____

Today I Feel...

Sleep Quality

Sleep Time

_____

Wake Time

_____

Date: _____

		Daily Servings	Hunger / Cravings

Whole Grains ☐ ☐ ☐ ☐

Beans & Legumes ☐ ☐ ☐

Berries ☐ ☐

Other Fruits ☐ ☐

Greens ☐ ☐

Cruciferous Vegetables ☐

Other Vegetables ☐

Flaxseed & Walnuts ☐

Other Nuts & Seeds ☐

Daily Servings

Hunger / Cravings

Some

None

Intense

Hydration

My Favorite Meal / Recipe Today Was:

_____
_____
_____
_____
_____

Today's Weight

Notes / My Important Numbers:

_____
_____
_____
_____
_____
_____
_____
_____

Today I Feel...

Sleep Quality

Sleep Time

_____

Wake Time

_____

Date: _____

Daily Servings

🌾 Whole Grains	☐ ☐ ☐ ☐
🫘 Beans & Legumes	☐ ☐ ☐
🍓 Berries	☐ ☐
🍎 Other Fruits	☐ ☐
🥬 Greens	☐ ☐
🥦 Cruciferous Vegetables	☐
🥕 Other Vegetables	☐
🌰 Flaxseed & Walnuts	☐
🥜 Other Nuts & Seeds	☐

Hunger / Cravings

None — Some — Intense

Hydration

My Favorite Meal / Recipe Today Was:

_____

_____

_____

_____

Today's Weight

Notes / My Important Numbers:

_____

_____

_____

_____

_____

_____

_____

Today I Feel...

Sleep Quality

Sleep Time

_____

Wake Time

_____

Date: _____

	Daily Servings	Hunger / Cravings

Whole Grains ☐ ☐ ☐ ☐

Beans & Legumes ☐ ☐ ☐

Berries ☐ ☐

Other Fruits ☐ ☐

Greens ☐ ☐

Cruciferous Vegetables ☐

Other Vegetables ☐

Flaxseed & Walnuts ☐

Other Nuts & Seeds ☐

Hunger / Cravings

Some

None   Intense

Hydration

My Favorite Meal / Recipe Today Was:

_____

_____

_____

_____

_____

Today's Weight

Notes / My Important Numbers:

_____

_____

_____

_____

_____

_____

_____

_____

Today I Feel...

Sleep Quality

Sleep Time

_____

Wake Time

_____

Date: _____

		Daily Servings

Whole Grains ☐ ☐ ☐ ☐

Beans & Legumes ☐ ☐ ☐

Berries ☐ ☐

Other Fruits ☐ ☐

Greens ☐ ☐

Cruciferous Vegetables ☐

Other Vegetables ☐

Flaxseed & Walnuts ☐

Other Nuts & Seeds ☐

Hunger / Cravings

Some

None — Intense

Hydration

My Favorite Meal / Recipe Today Was:

_____
_____
_____
_____
_____

Today's Weight

Notes / My Important Numbers:

_____
_____
_____
_____
_____
_____
_____

Today I Feel...

Sleep Quality

Sleep Time

_____

Wake Time

_____

Date: _____

Daily Servings

🌾 Whole Grains	☐ ☐ ☐ ☐
🫘 Beans & Legumes	☐ ☐ ☐
🍓 Berries	☐ ☐
🍐 Other Fruits	☐ ☐
🥦 Greens	☐ ☐
🥦 Cruciferous Vegetables	☐
🥕 Other Vegetables	☐
🌰 Flaxseed & Walnuts	☐
🥜 Other Nuts & Seeds	☐

Hunger / Cravings

None — Some — Intense

Hydration

My Favorite Meal / Recipe Today Was:

_____
_____
_____
_____
_____

Today's Weight

Notes / My Important Numbers:

_____
_____
_____
_____
_____
_____
_____

Today I Feel...

Sleep Quality

Sleep Time
_____

Wake Time
_____

Date: _____

		Daily Servings			
🌾	Whole Grains	☐	☐	☐	☐
🫘	Beans & Legumes	☐	☐	☐	
🍓	Berries	☐	☐		
🍐	Other Fruits	☐	☐		
🥬	Greens	☐	☐		
🥦	Cruciferous Vegetables	☐			
	Other Vegetables	☐			
	Flaxseed & Walnuts	☐			
	Other Nuts & Seeds	☐			

Hunger / Cravings

Some

None   Intense

Hydration

My Favorite Meal / Recipe Today Was:

_____

_____

_____

_____

Today's Weight

Notes / My Important Numbers:

_____

_____

_____

_____

_____

_____

_____

Today I Feel...

Sleep Quality

Sleep Time

_____

Wake Time

_____

z z z

Date: _____

		Daily Servings
🌾	Whole Grains	☐ ☐ ☐ ☐
🫘	Beans & Legumes	☐ ☐ ☐
🍓	Berries	☐ ☐
🍐	Other Fruits	☐ ☐
🥦	Greens	☐ ☐
🥦	Cruciferous Vegetables	☐
🌿	Other Vegetables	☐
🌰	Flaxseed & Walnuts	☐
🥜	Other Nuts & Seeds	☐

Hunger / Cravings

Some

None   Intense

Hydration

My Favorite Meal / Recipe Today Was:

_____
_____
_____
_____
_____

Today's Weight

Notes / My Important Numbers:

_____
_____
_____
_____
_____
_____
_____

Today I Feel...

Sleep Quality

Sleep Time

_____

Wake Time

_____

Date: _____

		Daily Servings
🌾	Whole Grains	☐ ☐ ☐ ☐
🫘	Beans & Legumes	☐ ☐ ☐
🍓	Berries	☐ ☐
🍑	Other Fruits	☐ ☐
🥬	Greens	☐ ☐
🥦	Cruciferous Vegetables	☐
	Other Vegetables	☐
	Flaxseed & Walnuts	☐
	Other Nuts & Seeds	☐

Hunger / Cravings

Some
None   Intense

Hydration

My Favorite Meal / Recipe Today Was:

_____

_____

_____

_____

Today's Weight

Notes / My Important Numbers:

_____

_____

_____

_____

_____

_____

_____

Today I Feel...

Sleep Quality

Sleep Time

_____

Wake Time

_____

Date: _____

Daily Servings

		Daily Servings

🌾 Whole Grains   ☐ ☐ ☐ ☐

🫘 Beans & Legumes   ☐ ☐ ☐

🍓 Berries   ☐ ☐

🍐 Other Fruits   ☐ ☐

🥦 Greens   ☐ ☐

🥦 Cruciferous Vegetables   ☐

🥬 Other Vegetables   ☐

🌰 Flaxseed & Walnuts   ☐

🥜 Other Nuts & Seeds   ☐

Hunger / Cravings

None — Some — Intense

Hydration

My Favorite Meal / Recipe Today Was:

_____
_____
_____
_____
_____

Today's Weight

Notes / My Important Numbers:

_____
_____
_____
_____
_____
_____
_____

Today I Feel...

Sleep Quality

Sleep Time

_____

Wake Time

_____

Date: _____

		Daily Servings

Whole Grains ☐ ☐ ☐ ☐

Beans & Legumes ☐ ☐ ☐

Berries ☐ ☐

Other Fruits ☐ ☐

Greens ☐ ☐

Cruciferous Vegetables ☐

Other Vegetables ☐

Flaxseed & Walnuts ☐

Other Nuts & Seeds ☐

Hunger / Cravings

Some

None   Intense

Hydration

My Favorite Meal / Recipe Today Was:

_____

_____

_____

_____

_____

Today's Weight

Notes / My Important Numbers:

_____

_____

_____

_____

_____

_____

_____

Today I Feel...

Sleep Quality

Sleep Time

_____

Wake Time

_____

Date: _____

		Daily Servings	Hunger / Cravings

Whole Grains   ☐ ☐ ☐ ☐

Beans & Legumes   ☐ ☐ ☐

Berries   ☐ ☐

Other Fruits   ☐ ☐

Greens   ☐ ☐

Cruciferous Vegetables   ☐

Other Vegetables   ☐

Flaxseed & Walnuts   ☐

Other Nuts & Seeds   ☐

Hunger / Cravings

Some

None   Intense

Hydration

My Favorite Meal / Recipe Today Was:

_____

_____

_____

_____

_____

Today's Weight

Notes / My Important Numbers:

_____

_____

_____

_____

_____

_____

_____

_____

Today I Feel...

Sleep Quality

Sleep Time

_____

Wake Time

_____

Date: _____

		Daily Servings

Whole Grains ☐ ☐ ☐ ☐

Beans & Legumes ☐ ☐ ☐

Berries ☐ ☐

Other Fruits ☐ ☐

Greens ☐ ☐

Cruciferous Vegetables ☐

Other Vegetables ☐

Flaxseed & Walnuts ☐

Other Nuts & Seeds ☐

Hunger / Cravings

Some

None — Intense

Hydration

My Favorite Meal / Recipe Today Was:

_____

_____

_____

_____

Today's Weight

Notes / My Important Numbers:

_____

_____

_____

_____

_____

_____

_____

_____

Today I Feel...

Sleep Quality

Sleep Time

_____

Wake Time

_____

Date: _____

Daily Servings	Hunger / Cravings

🌾 Whole Grains   ☐ ☐ ☐ ☐

🫘 Beans & Legumes   ☐ ☐ ☐

🍓 Berries   ☐ ☐

🍐 Other Fruits   ☐ ☐

🥬 Greens   ☐ ☐

🥦 Cruciferous Vegetables   ☐

🧅 Other Vegetables   ☐

🌰 Flaxseed & Walnuts   ☐

🥜 Other Nuts & Seeds   ☐

Hunger / Cravings

Some
None — Intense

Hydration

My Favorite Meal / Recipe Today Was:

_____

_____

_____

_____

_____

Today's Weight

Notes / My Important Numbers:

_____

_____

_____

_____

_____

_____

_____

Today I Feel...

Sleep Quality

Sleep Time

_____

Wake Time

_____

Date: _____

Daily Servings

🌾 Whole Grains	☐ ☐ ☐ ☐
🫘 Beans & Legumes	☐ ☐ ☐
🍓 Berries	☐ ☐
🍐 Other Fruits	☐ ☐
🥬 Greens	☐ ☐
🥦 Cruciferous Vegetables	☐
🥕 Other Vegetables	☐
🌰 Flaxseed & Walnuts	☐
🥜 Other Nuts & Seeds	☐

Hunger / Cravings

Some

None — Intense

Hydration

My Favorite Meal / Recipe Today Was:

_____
_____
_____
_____

Today's Weight

Notes / My Important Numbers:

_____
_____
_____
_____
_____
_____

Today I Feel...

Sleep Quality

Sleep Time

_____

Wake Time

_____

Date: _____

	Daily Servings	Hunger / Cravings

Whole Grains ☐ ☐ ☐ ☐

Beans & Legumes ☐ ☐ ☐

Berries ☐ ☐

Other Fruits ☐ ☐

Greens ☐ ☐

Cruciferous Vegetables ☐

Other Vegetables ☐

Flaxseed & Walnuts ☐

Other Nuts & Seeds ☐

Hunger / Cravings

Some

None

Intense

Hydration

My Favorite Meal / Recipe Today Was:

_____

_____

_____

_____

_____

Today's Weight

Notes / My Important Numbers:

_____

_____

_____

_____

_____

_____

_____

_____

Today I Feel...

Sleep Quality

Sleep Time

_____

Wake Time

_____

Date: _____

		Daily Servings	Hunger / Cravings

Whole Grains ☐ ☐ ☐ ☐

Beans & Legumes ☐ ☐ ☐

Berries ☐ ☐

Other Fruits ☐ ☐

Greens ☐ ☐

Cruciferous Vegetables ☐

Other Vegetables ☐

Flaxseed & Walnuts ☐

Other Nuts & Seeds ☐

Daily Servings

Hunger / Cravings

Some

None — Intense

Hydration

My Favorite Meal / Recipe Today Was:

_____
_____
_____
_____
_____

Today's Weight

Notes / My Important Numbers:

_____
_____
_____
_____
_____
_____
_____

Today I Feel...

Sleep Quality

Sleep Time

_____

Wake Time

_____

Date: _____

Whole Grains

Beans & Legumes

Berries

Other Fruits

Greens

Cruciferous Vegetables

Other Vegetables

Flaxseed & Walnuts

Other Nuts & Seeds

Hunger / Cravings

Some

None

Intense

Hydration

My Favorite Meal / Recipe Today Was:

_____

_____

_____

_____

_____

Today's Weight

Notes / My Important Numbers:

_____

_____

_____

_____

_____

_____

_____

_____

Today I Feel...

Sleep Quality

Sleep Time

_____

Wake Time

_____

Date: _____

Daily Servings

🌾 Whole Grains ☐ ☐ ☐ ☐

🫘 Beans & Legumes ☐ ☐ ☐

🍓 Berries ☐ ☐

🍐 Other Fruits ☐ ☐

🥬 Greens ☐ ☐

🥦 Cruciferous Vegetables ☐

🫚 Other Vegetables ☐

🌰 Flaxseed & Walnuts ☐

🥜 Other Nuts & Seeds ☐

Hunger / Cravings

Some

None — Intense

Hydration

My Favorite Meal / Recipe Today Was:

_____

_____

_____

_____

_____

Today's Weight

Notes / My Important Numbers:

_____

_____

_____

_____

_____

_____

_____

_____

Today I Feel...

Sleep Quality

Sleep Time

_____

Wake Time

_____

Date: _____

		Daily Servings

Whole Grains ☐ ☐ ☐ ☐

Beans & Legumes ☐ ☐ ☐

Berries ☐ ☐

Other Fruits ☐ ☐

Greens ☐ ☐

Cruciferous Vegetables ☐

Other Vegetables ☐

Flaxseed & Walnuts ☐

Other Nuts & Seeds ☐

Hunger / Cravings

Some

None — Intense

Hydration

My Favorite Meal / Recipe Today Was:

_____

_____

_____

_____

_____

Today's Weight

Notes / My Important Numbers:

_____

_____

_____

_____

_____

_____

_____

Today I Feel...

Sleep Quality

Sleep Time

_____

Wake Time

_____

Date: _____

		Daily Servings	Hunger / Cravings

Whole Grains ☐ ☐ ☐ ☐

Beans & Legumes ☐ ☐ ☐

Berries ☐ ☐

Other Fruits ☐ ☐

Greens ☐ ☐

Cruciferous Vegetables ☐

Other Vegetables ☐

Flaxseed & Walnuts ☐

Other Nuts & Seeds ☐

Daily Servings

Hunger / Cravings

Some
None — Intense

Hydration

My Favorite Meal / Recipe Today Was:

_____

_____

_____

_____

_____

Today's Weight

Notes / My Important Numbers:

_____

_____

_____

_____

_____

_____

_____

Today I Feel...

Sleep Quality

Sleep Time

_____

Wake Time

_____

Date: _____

Daily Servings

🌾 Whole Grains	☐ ☐ ☐ ☐
🫘 Beans & Legumes	☐ ☐ ☐
🍓 Berries	☐ ☐
🍏 Other Fruits	☐ ☐
🥦 Greens	☐ ☐
🥦 Cruciferous Vegetables	☐
🍅 Other Vegetables	☐
🌰 Flaxseed & Walnuts	☐
🥜 Other Nuts & Seeds	☐

Hunger / Cravings

None — Some — Intense

Hydration

My Favorite Meal / Recipe Today Was:

_____

_____

_____

_____

_____

Today's Weight

Notes / My Important Numbers:

_____

_____

_____

_____

_____

_____

_____

_____

Today I Feel...

Sleep Quality

Sleep Time

_____

Wake Time

_____

Date: _____

		Daily Servings
🌾	Whole Grains	☐ ☐ ☐ ☐
🫘	Beans & Legumes	☐ ☐ ☐
🍓	Berries	☐ ☐
🍑	Other Fruits	☐ ☐
🥦	Greens	☐ ☐
🥦	Cruciferous Vegetables	☐
	Other Vegetables	☐
	Flaxseed & Walnuts	☐
🥜	Other Nuts & Seeds	☐

Hunger / Cravings

Some
None   Intense

Hydration

My Favorite Meal / Recipe Today Was:

_____
_____
_____
_____

Today's Weight

Notes / My Important Numbers:

_____
_____
_____
_____
_____
_____
_____

Today I Feel...

Sleep Quality

Sleep Time

_____

Wake Time

_____

Date: _____

Daily Servings

Food	Servings
🌾 Whole Grains	☐ ☐ ☐ ☐
🫘 Beans & Legumes	☐ ☐ ☐
🍓 Berries	☐ ☐
🍐 Other Fruits	☐ ☐
🥬 Greens	☐ ☐
🥦 Cruciferous Vegetables	☐
🥕 Other Vegetables	☐
🌰 Flaxseed & Walnuts	☐
🥜 Other Nuts & Seeds	☐

Hunger / Cravings

Some

None / Intense

Hydration

My Favorite Meal / Recipe Today Was:

_____
_____
_____
_____
_____

Today's Weight

Notes / My Important Numbers:

_____
_____
_____
_____
_____
_____
_____

Today I Feel...

Sleep Quality

Sleep Time

_____

Wake Time

_____

Date: _____

| Daily Servings | | Hunger / Cravings |

🌾 Whole Grains	☐ ☐ ☐ ☐	
🫘 Beans & Legumes	☐ ☐ ☐	
🍓 Berries	☐ ☐	
🍑 Other Fruits	☐ ☐	
🥬 Greens	☐ ☐	
🥦 Cruciferous Vegetables	☐	
🍆 Other Vegetables	☐	
🌰 Flaxseed & Walnuts	☐	
🥜 Other Nuts & Seeds	☐	

Hunger / Cravings

Some — None — Intense

Hydration

My Favorite Meal / Recipe Today Was:

_____

_____

_____

_____

Today's Weight

Notes / My Important Numbers:

_____

_____

_____

_____

_____

_____

_____

_____

Today I Feel...

Sleep Quality

Sleep Time

_____

Wake Time

_____

Date: _____

		Daily Servings	Hunger / Cravings

Whole Grains ☐ ☐ ☐ ☐

Beans & Legumes ☐ ☐ ☐

Berries ☐ ☐

Other Fruits ☐ ☐

Greens ☐ ☐

Cruciferous Vegetables ☐

Other Vegetables ☐

Flaxseed & Walnuts ☐

Other Nuts & Seeds ☐

Daily Servings

Hunger / Cravings

Some

None

Intense

Hydration

My Favorite Meal / Recipe Today Was:

_____

_____

_____

_____

_____

Today's Weight

Notes / My Important Numbers:

Today I Feel...

_____

_____

_____

_____

_____

_____

_____

Sleep Quality

Sleep Time

_____

Wake Time

_____

Date: _____

Daily Servings

🌾 Whole Grains	☐ ☐ ☐ ☐	
🫘 Beans & Legumes	☐ ☐ ☐	
🍓 Berries	☐ ☐	
🍎 Other Fruits	☐ ☐	
🥦 Greens	☐ ☐	
🥦 Cruciferous Vegetables	☐	
🥕 Other Vegetables	☐	
🌰 Flaxseed & Walnuts	☐	
🥜 Other Nuts & Seeds	☐	

Hunger / Cravings

Some

None — Intense

Hydration

My Favorite Meal / Recipe Today Was:

_____
_____
_____
_____
_____

Today's Weight

Notes / My Important Numbers:

_____
_____
_____
_____
_____
_____
_____
_____

Today I Feel...

Sleep Quality

Sleep Time

_____

Wake Time

_____

Date: _____

		Daily Servings	Hunger / Cravings

Whole Grains ☐ ☐ ☐ ☐

Beans & Legumes ☐ ☐ ☐

Berries ☐ ☐

Other Fruits ☐ ☐

Greens ☐ ☐

Cruciferous Vegetables ☐

Other Vegetables ☐

Flaxseed & Walnuts ☐

Other Nuts & Seeds ☐

Daily Servings

Hunger / Cravings

Some
None · Intense

Hydration

My Favorite Meal / Recipe Today Was:

_____

_____

_____

_____

_____

Today's Weight

Notes / My Important Numbers:

_____

_____

_____

_____

_____

_____

_____

_____

Today I Feel...

Sleep Quality

Sleep Time

_____

Wake Time

_____

Date: _____

Whole Grains

Beans & Legumes

Berries

Other Fruits

Greens

Cruciferous Vegetables

Other Vegetables

Flaxseed & Walnuts

Other Nuts & Seeds

Daily Servings
☐ ☐ ☐ ☐
☐ ☐ ☐
☐ ☐
☐ ☐
☐ ☐
☐
☐
☐
☐

Hunger / Cravings

Some

None

Intense

Hydration

My Favorite Meal / Recipe Today Was:

_____

_____

_____

_____

Today's Weight

Notes / My Important Numbers:

_____

_____

_____

_____

_____

_____

_____

Today I Feel...

Sleep Quality

Sleep Time

_____

Wake Time

_____

Date: _____

		Daily Servings	Hunger / Cravings

Whole Grains ☐ ☐ ☐ ☐

Beans & Legumes ☐ ☐ ☐

Berries ☐ ☐

Other Fruits ☐ ☐

Greens ☐ ☐

Cruciferous Vegetables ☐

Other Vegetables ☐

Flaxseed & Walnuts ☐

Other Nuts & Seeds ☐

Daily Servings

Hunger / Cravings

Some

None   Intense

Hydration

My Favorite Meal / Recipe Today Was:

_____

_____

_____

_____

_____

Today's Weight

Notes / My Important Numbers:

Today I Feel...

_____

_____

_____

_____

_____

_____

_____

Sleep Quality

Sleep Time

_____

Wake Time

_____

Date: _____

		Daily Servings
🌾	Whole Grains	☐ ☐ ☐ ☐
🫘	Beans & Legumes	☐ ☐ ☐
🍓	Berries	☐ ☐
🍐	Other Fruits	☐ ☐
🥦	Greens	☐ ☐
🥦	Cruciferous Vegetables	☐
🍆	Other Vegetables	☐
🌰	Flaxseed & Walnuts	☐
🥜	Other Nuts & Seeds	☐

Hunger / Cravings

Some

None — Intense

Hydration

My Favorite Meal / Recipe Today Was:

_____
_____
_____
_____

Today's Weight

Notes / My Important Numbers:

_____
_____
_____
_____
_____
_____
_____

Today I Feel...

Sleep Quality

Sleep Time

_____

Wake Time

_____

Date: _____

	Daily Servings	Hunger / Cravings

Whole Grains ☐ ☐ ☐ ☐

Beans & Legumes ☐ ☐ ☐

Berries ☐ ☐

Other Fruits ☐ ☐

Greens ☐ ☐

Cruciferous Vegetables ☐

Other Vegetables ☐

Flaxseed & Walnuts ☐

Other Nuts & Seeds ☐

Hunger / Cravings

Some · None · Intense

Hydration

My Favorite Meal / Recipe Today Was:

_____

_____

_____

_____

_____

Today's Weight

Notes / My Important Numbers:

_____

_____

_____

_____

_____

_____

Today I Feel...

Sleep Quality

Sleep Time

_____

Wake Time

_____

Date: _____

Daily Servings

🌾 Whole Grains	☐ ☐ ☐ ☐
🫘 Beans & Legumes	☐ ☐ ☐
🍓 Berries	☐ ☐
🍐 Other Fruits	☐ ☐
🥦 Greens	☐ ☐
🥦 Cruciferous Vegetables	☐
🥗 Other Vegetables	☐
🌰 Flaxseed & Walnuts	☐
Other Nuts & Seeds	☐

Hunger / Cravings

Some
None — Intense

Hydration

My Favorite Meal / Recipe Today Was:

_____
_____
_____
_____
_____

Today's Weight

Notes / My Important Numbers:

_____
_____
_____
_____
_____
_____
_____

Today I Feel...

Sleep Quality

Sleep Time
_____

Wake Time
_____

Date: _____

Daily Servings

🌾 Whole Grains	☐ ☐ ☐ ☐	
🫘 Beans & Legumes	☐ ☐ ☐	
🍓 Berries	☐ ☐	
🍐 Other Fruits	☐ ☐	
🥬 Greens	☐ ☐	
🥦 Cruciferous Vegetables	☐	
🥗 Other Vegetables	☐	
🌰 Flaxseed & Walnuts	☐	
🥜 Other Nuts & Seeds	☐	

Hunger / Cravings

Some

None — Intense

Hydration

My Favorite Meal / Recipe Today Was:

_____

_____

_____

_____

Today's Weight

Notes / My Important Numbers:

_____

_____

_____

_____

_____

_____

_____

Today I Feel...

Sleep Quality

Sleep Time

_____

Wake Time

_____

Date: _____

	Daily Servings	
🌾 Whole Grains	☐ ☐ ☐ ☐	
🫘 Beans & Legumes	☐ ☐ ☐	
🍓 Berries	☐ ☐	
🍐 Other Fruits	☐ ☐	
🥦 Greens	☐ ☐	
🥦 Cruciferous Vegetables	☐	
🌱 Other Vegetables	☐	
🌰 Flaxseed & Walnuts	☐	
🌰 Other Nuts & Seeds	☐	

Hunger / Cravings

Hydration

My Favorite Meal / Recipe Today Was:

_____
_____
_____
_____
_____

Today's Weight

Notes / My Important Numbers:

_____
_____
_____
_____
_____
_____
_____
_____

Today I Feel...

Sleep Quality

Sleep Time

_____

Wake Time

_____

Date: _____

		Daily Servings	Hunger / Cravings

Daily Servings

🌾 Whole Grains ☐ ☐ ☐ ☐

🫘 Beans & Legumes ☐ ☐ ☐

🍓 Berries ☐ ☐

🍐 Other Fruits ☐ ☐

🥦 Greens ☐ ☐

🥦 Cruciferous Vegetables ☐

🧅 Other Vegetables ☐

🌰 Flaxseed & Walnuts ☐

🥜 Other Nuts & Seeds ☐

Hunger / Cravings

Some

None / Intense

Hydration

My Favorite Meal / Recipe Today Was:

_____
_____
_____
_____
_____

Today's Weight

Notes / My Important Numbers:

_____
_____
_____
_____
_____
_____
_____
_____

Today I Feel...

Sleep Quality

Sleep Time

_____

Wake Time

_____

Date: _____

		Daily Servings			

Whole Grains   ☐ ☐ ☐ ☐

Beans & Legumes   ☐ ☐ ☐

Berries   ☐ ☐

Other Fruits   ☐ ☐

Greens   ☐ ☐

Cruciferous Vegetables   ☐

Other Vegetables   ☐

Flaxseed & Walnuts   ☐

Other Nuts & Seeds   ☐

Hunger / Cravings

Some
None   Intense

Hydration

My Favorite Meal / Recipe Today Was:

_____

_____

_____

_____

_____

Today's Weight

Notes / My Important Numbers:

_____

_____

_____

_____

_____

_____

_____

Today I Feel...

Sleep Quality

Sleep Time

_____

Wake Time

_____

Date: _____

	Daily Servings	Hunger / Cravings

Whole Grains ☐ ☐ ☐ ☐

Beans & Legumes ☐ ☐ ☐

Berries ☐ ☐

Other Fruits ☐ ☐

Greens ☐ ☐

Cruciferous Vegetables ☐

Other Vegetables ☐

Flaxseed & Walnuts ☐

Other Nuts & Seeds ☐

Hunger / Cravings

Some / None / Intense

Hydration

My Favorite Meal / Recipe Today Was:

_____

_____

_____

_____

_____

Today's Weight

Notes / My Important Numbers:

_____

_____

_____

_____

_____

_____

_____

_____

Today I Feel...

Sleep Quality

Sleep Time

_____

Wake Time

_____

Date: _____

		Daily Servings

Whole Grains ☐ ☐ ☐ ☐

Beans & Legumes ☐ ☐ ☐

Berries ☐ ☐

Other Fruits ☐ ☐

Greens ☐ ☐

Cruciferous Vegetables ☐

Other Vegetables ☐

Flaxseed & Walnuts ☐

Other Nuts & Seeds ☐

Hunger / Cravings

Some
None / Intense

Hydration

My Favorite Meal / Recipe Today Was:

_____
_____
_____
_____

Today's Weight

Notes / My Important Numbers:

_____
_____
_____
_____
_____
_____
_____

Today I Feel...

Sleep Quality

Sleep Time

_____

Wake Time

_____

Date: _____

Daily Servings

Whole Grains	☐ ☐ ☐ ☐
Beans & Legumes	☐ ☐ ☐
Berries	☐ ☐
Other Fruits	☐ ☐
Greens	☐ ☐
Cruciferous Vegetables	☐
Other Vegetables	☐
Flaxseed & Walnuts	☐
Other Nuts & Seeds	☐

Hunger / Cravings

Some
None
Intense

Hydration

My Favorite Meal / Recipe Today Was:

_____
_____
_____
_____
_____

Today's Weight

Notes / My Important Numbers:

_____
_____
_____
_____
_____
_____
_____

Today I Feel...

Sleep Quality

Sleep Time

_____

Wake Time

_____

Date: _____

		Daily Servings			

Whole Grains ☐ ☐ ☐ ☐

Beans & Legumes ☐ ☐ ☐

Berries ☐ ☐

Other Fruits ☐ ☐

Greens ☐ ☐

Cruciferous Vegetables ☐

Other Vegetables ☐

Flaxseed & Walnuts ☐

Other Nuts & Seeds ☐

Hunger / Cravings

Some

None   Intense

Hydration

My Favorite Meal / Recipe Today Was:

_____

_____

_____

_____

Today's Weight

Notes / My Important Numbers:

_____

_____

_____

_____

_____

_____

_____

Today I Feel...

Sleep Quality

Sleep Time

_____

Wake Time

_____

Date: _____

Daily Servings

Whole Grains ☐ ☐ ☐ ☐
Beans & Legumes ☐ ☐ ☐
Berries ☐ ☐
Other Fruits ☐ ☐
Greens ☐ ☐
Cruciferous Vegetables ☐
Other Vegetables ☐
Flaxseed & Walnuts ☐
Other Nuts & Seeds ☐

Hunger / Cravings

Some
None
Intense

Hydration

My Favorite Meal / Recipe Today Was:

_____
_____
_____
_____
_____

Today's Weight

Notes / My Important Numbers:

_____
_____
_____
_____
_____
_____
_____

Today I Feel...

Sleep Quality

Sleep Time
_____

Wake Time
_____

Date: _____

		Daily Servings	Hunger / Cravings

Whole Grains ☐ ☐ ☐ ☐

Beans & Legumes ☐ ☐ ☐

Berries ☐ ☐

Other Fruits ☐ ☐

Greens ☐ ☐

Cruciferous Vegetables ☐

Other Vegetables ☐

Flaxseed & Walnuts ☐

Other Nuts & Seeds ☐

Hunger / Cravings

None — Some — Intense

Hydration

My Favorite Meal / Recipe Today Was:

_____

_____

_____

_____

_____

Today's Weight

Notes / My Important Numbers:

_____

_____

_____

_____

_____

_____

_____

Today I Feel...

Sleep Quality

Sleep Time

_____

Wake Time

_____

Date: _____

		Daily Servings	Hunger / Cravings

Daily Servings

Whole Grains ☐ ☐ ☐ ☐

Beans & Legumes ☐ ☐ ☐

Berries ☐ ☐

Other Fruits ☐ ☐

Greens ☐ ☐

Cruciferous Vegetables ☐

Other Vegetables ☐

Flaxseed & Walnuts ☐

Other Nuts & Seeds ☐

Hunger / Cravings

Some

None   Intense

Hydration

My Favorite Meal / Recipe Today Was:

_____

_____

_____

_____

_____

Today's Weight

Notes / My Important Numbers:

_____

_____

_____

_____

_____

_____

_____

Today I Feel...

Sleep Quality

Sleep Time

_____

Wake Time

_____

Date: _____

		Daily Servings			

Whole Grains ☐ ☐ ☐ ☐

Beans & Legumes ☐ ☐ ☐

Berries ☐ ☐

Other Fruits ☐ ☐

Greens ☐ ☐

Cruciferous Vegetables ☐

Other Vegetables ☐

Flaxseed & Walnuts ☐

Other Nuts & Seeds ☐

Hunger / Cravings

Some
None
Intense

Hydration

My Favorite Meal / Recipe Today Was:

_____
_____
_____
_____
_____

Today's Weight

Notes / My Important Numbers:

_____
_____
_____
_____
_____
_____
_____
_____

Today I Feel...

Sleep Quality

Sleep Time

_____

Wake Time

_____

Date: _____

		Daily Servings				Hunger / Cravings

Whole Grains ☐ ☐ ☐ ☐

Beans & Legumes ☐ ☐ ☐

Berries ☐ ☐

Other Fruits ☐ ☐

Greens ☐ ☐

Cruciferous Vegetables ☐

Other Vegetables ☐

Flaxseed & Walnuts ☐

Other Nuts & Seeds ☐

Daily Servings

Hunger / Cravings

Some

None

Intense

Hydration

My Favorite Meal / Recipe Today Was:

_____

_____

_____

_____

_____

Today's Weight

Notes / My Important Numbers:

_____

_____

_____

_____

_____

_____

_____

Today I Feel...

Sleep Quality

Sleep Time

_____

Wake Time

_____

Date: _____

		Daily Servings	Hunger / Cravings

Whole Grains ☐ ☐ ☐ ☐

Beans & Legumes ☐ ☐ ☐

Berries ☐ ☐

Other Fruits ☐ ☐

Greens ☐ ☐

Cruciferous Vegetables ☐

Other Vegetables ☐

Flaxseed & Walnuts ☐

Other Nuts & Seeds ☐

Daily Servings

Hunger / Cravings

Some

None — Intense

Hydration

My Favorite Meal / Recipe Today Was:

_____

_____

_____

_____

Today's Weight

Notes / My Important Numbers:

_____

_____

_____

_____

_____

_____

_____

Today I Feel...

Sleep Quality

Sleep Time

_____

Wake Time

_____

Date: _____

		Daily Servings	Hunger / Cravings

Daily Servings

Hunger / Cravings

🌾 Whole Grains ☐ ☐ ☐ ☐

🫘 Beans & Legumes ☐ ☐ ☐

🍓 Berries ☐ ☐

🍐 Other Fruits ☐ ☐

🥦 Greens ☐ ☐

🥦 Cruciferous Vegetables ☐

🥗 Other Vegetables ☐

🌰 Flaxseed & Walnuts ☐

🥜 Other Nuts & Seeds ☐

Hydration

My Favorite Meal / Recipe Today Was:

_____
_____
_____
_____
_____

Today's Weight

Notes / My Important Numbers:

_____
_____
_____
_____
_____
_____
_____

Today I Feel...

Sleep Quality

Sleep Time

_____

Wake Time

_____

Date: _____

		Daily Servings			

Whole Grains ☐ ☐ ☐ ☐

Beans & Legumes ☐ ☐ ☐

Berries ☐ ☐

Other Fruits ☐ ☐

Greens ☐ ☐

Cruciferous Vegetables ☐

Other Vegetables ☐

Flaxseed & Walnuts ☐

Other Nuts & Seeds ☐

Hunger / Cravings

Some

None — Intense

Hydration

My Favorite Meal / Recipe Today Was:

_____

_____

_____

_____

Today's Weight

Notes / My Important Numbers:

_____

_____

_____

_____

_____

_____

_____

Today I Feel...

Sleep Quality

Sleep Time

_____

Wake Time

_____

Date: _____

	Daily Servings

Whole Grains ☐ ☐ ☐ ☐

Beans & Legumes ☐ ☐ ☐

Berries ☐ ☐

Other Fruits ☐ ☐

Greens ☐ ☐

Cruciferous Vegetables ☐

Other Vegetables ☐

Flaxseed & Walnuts ☐

Other Nuts & Seeds ☐

Hunger / Cravings

Some

None

Intense

Hydration

My Favorite Meal / Recipe Today Was:

_____

_____

_____

_____

_____

Today's Weight

Notes / My Important Numbers:

_____

_____

_____

_____

_____

_____

_____

Today I Feel...

Sleep Quality

Sleep Time

_____

Wake Time

_____

Printed in Great Britain
by Amazon

35494078R00059